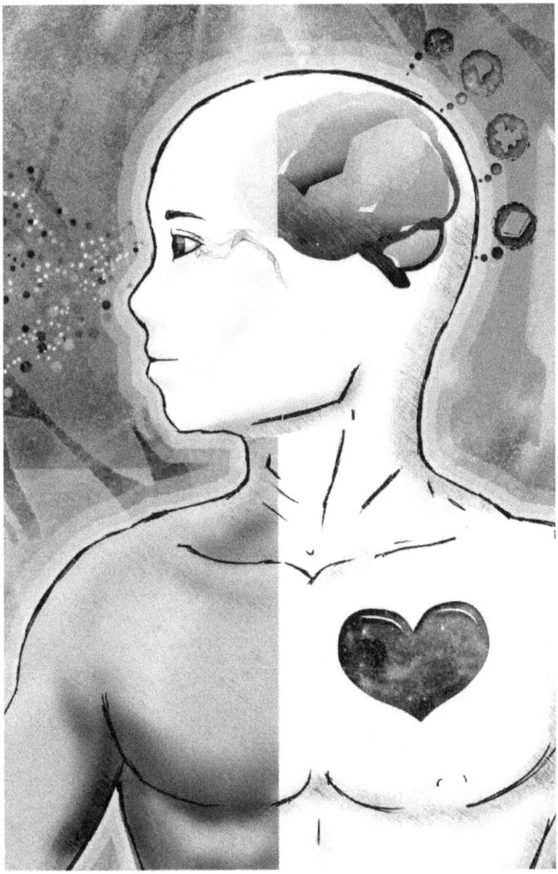

Body Empowerment

BODY EMPOWERMENT

Body Empowerment

BODY EMPOWERMENT

Unearth the Force of Your Body

Instafo

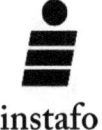

instafo

ISBN 978-1-542-71854-7

Printed in the United States of America

First Edition

CONTENTS

Chapter 1: Empowering the Body

1.1 More Than Fresh and Blood.......................................11

1.2 The Human Battery...12

1.3 Activity: Start Engine Right.......................................15

Chapter 2: Filtering the Body

2.1 To Go Organic, or Not to Go Organic......................17

2.2 Label Matters..20

2.3 Exercise: Spring Clean..23

Chapter 3: Fueling the Body

3.1 Outdated Eating Machine..25

3.2 The One-Third Meal Plan...26

3.3 Portion Eating..31

3.4 Exercise: Update Eating Machine.............................34

Chapter 4: Exercising the Body

4.1 Workout Simplified..35

4.2 Types of Exercises...36

4.3 Physical Activities Schedule.......................39

4.4 Exercise: Choose Workouts........................42

Chapter 5: Rejuvenating the Body

5.1 Recharge Session...43

5.2 Pre-SLEEP-Quisites.....................................44

5.3 Applying the Rules of Sleep........................47

Chapter 6: Redesigning the Body

6.1 Exercise 1: Know Organic...........................51

6.2 Exercise 2: Upgrade Meals.........................53

6.3 Exercise 3: Get Physical..............................54

6.4 Exercise 4: Prepare Rest..............................56

Chapter 7: Embracing the Powerful Body

7.1 Bodily Neglect...58

7.2 Bodily Perfect..59

Body Empowerment

Body Empowerment

Chapter 1:

Empowering the Body

More Than Fresh and Blood

To the majority of folks, the body is sadly seen as only a superficial shell through which we express our inner selves

Fortunately, we have all come a long way and have all heard in some shape or form the phrase, "It doesn't matter what you look like on the outside, it's what's on the inside that counts." Now while this is certainly a nice rule to live by, for many of us, expressions like these are simply excuses not to get ourselves in shape and most of all—healthy.

The truth is that your body is not just a human shell; it is more like an active conduit which processes everything we need to be strong and stay alive, such as vitamins, minerals and amino acids. Using these, our body carries out specific functions that, in turn, manifest themselves beneficially for us, such as experiencing a better mood, having greater energy, or simply being happier.

For this is the reason why you would want to empower your body.

The Human Battery

Empowering your body can be compared to charging a car's battery. It's what allows you to do everything one needs to do, whether it be physical or mental work.

Like a car's battery that needs to be recharged after too much use, the human body needs the proper "charge"—in this case, healthy food, exercise, and sleep—so that it can regain energy and function optimally.

Empowering your body shouldn't be about impressing anyone. Though, undoubtedly when one does take care of one's body there are going to be admirable attentions from others, but that shouldn't be the main goal. Body empowerment means getting and staying healthy, so you can live your best life.

- An empowered body will improve your health through making the right choices about what you eat and how you eat.

- An empowered body will present the perfect opportunity to finally be able to get in shape and look great.

- An empowered body will boost your confidence levels as a result of looking and feeling better about yourself.

Thus, empowering your body should be all about doing it for you, and no one else.

Activity: Start Engine Right

Before proceeding any further, here's an activity for you.

In the morning, after waking up, try this quick routine.

1. Don't eat right away. Right after waking up, describe, in a few words, your current energy levels, e.g., "I have no energy—I want to go back to bed immediately."

2. Set your timer for 10 minutes and begin running or walking, (whichever you prefer).

3. After you are done running or walking for the 10 minutes, have a glass of water and express how you feel, e.g., "My heart beat is fast now, but I actually feel more motivated than earlier."

This demonstration is supposed to show you how exercise can have a positive effect on your body and your mood.

Now that you have dabbled with this little experiment, let's move on.

<u>Chapter 2:</u>

Filtering the Body

To Go Organic, or Not to Go Organic

A simple trip to the grocery store can quickly become an anxiety-ridden experience when faced with the dizzying number of choices available.

Let's say you want an apple. Should you get the regular apple or the organic apple? The regular apple looks just as tasty as the organic apple, though the latter costs 3 times more! So you say to yourself, "Huh! Capitalism—what a tricky system! Isn't it?" You are certainly justified in feeling confused. The economic system is quite tricky.

Just as big corporations often eliminate jobs to maximize profits, they also jeopardize food safety in pursuit of the almighty dollar.

Specifically, we are referring to the chemically-enhanced food that we all eat every day.

Chemically-enhanced food, or genetically-engineered food (GMO), is food grown using pesticides or chemicals to kill insects, weeds and fungi that can often ruin crops. They also include cattle and other farm animals, which are given antibiotics or fed chemically-enriched grains.

Many of these methods are great for farmers and agricultural companies as they result in high-yield crops and increased production. However, many nutrition experts recommend choosing organic over chemically-enhanced foods (despite the increase in cost) for some of these following reasons:

- **To avoid any toxic chemical.** It should go without saying that chemically-enhanced food can be unhealthy for you because we don't know the long-term side effects from that chemical with all them out there. There are about 600 registered active chemicals used in food processes in the USA alone.

- **To provide better nutrition for your body.** Organic farming is held to a higher standard than traditional farming, including the use of soil that is cultivated with sustainable practices and is naturally fortified. This produces foods that have more enzymes, vitamins and micronutrients.

- **To reduce risk of developing diseases.** By going organic, you are avoiding food with pesticides and other foreign genetic materials. Organic food is required to be grown without the use of certain pesticides and fertilizers; and pesticides have been shown to cause diseases like cancer, neurological problems, and birth defects.

- **And lastly, to experience better taste.** Don't believe us? Try a blind taste-test with a fruit, and you'll see the difference. If you want a more flavorful meal, organic is the way to go. And who doesn't want to enjoy a healthier and tastier meal?

Label Matters

So the first step in creating total body empowerment is to know the difference between organic food and non-organic food.

Learn how to read the labeling on food packaging. Organic products are almost always clearly labeled as organic. When choosing non-organic items, scrutinize the label even more closely.

According to Mark Lorch, a lecturer in chemistry at the University of Hull (in Great Britain), there are some chemicals you should always avoid, like E290, 8-Methyl-N-vannillyl-6-nonenamide, Denatured protein, DHMO, NaCl, and Uranium.

If you see these chemicals on the list of ingredients of your favorite soda or cake mix, leave them on the shelf! Some of these chemicals, like NaCl (which is often used on salty snacks), are actually considered poisonous.

Lorch also states that denatured protein is linked to Alzheimer's disease, Parkinson's disease and Creutzfeldt-Jakob disease. So watch out for these ingredients and don't allow these chemicals into your home.

It's helpful to know the types of foods that are suspect to harboring some of these dangerous chemicals. They are normally found in products sold in large quantities and are, you guessed it—cheap.

When budgeting for food, it's best to spend the extra money on the organic version of the following products—

poultry, pork, beef, apples, pears, tomatoes, potatoes, spinach, coffee, peaches, nectarines, grapes, celery, red and green bell peppers, milk, cheese, butter, strawberries, cherries and raspberries.

The non-organic versions of these foods are either fed with antibiotics that remain in the meat or are sprayed with harmful insecticides. US regulations for protecting consumers from these harmful practices are quite lax, though efforts are being made to change these standards as more people become aware of the effects of these toxic chemicals.

So start your journey toward healthier living today, by clearing your fridge and pantry from all chemically-processed foods. It's never too late to rid yourself of all the junk and start making better choices.

Exercise: Spring Clean

To kick things off, let's get started on the following exercise:

1. Go through your kitchen items and look for ingredients that are considered harmful or too hard to pronounce and make a decision to ban them from your kitchen completely. Remember that if these items don't make it into your kitchen in the first place, then they won't be eaten!

2. Look for a local grocery store with a special section for organic fruits, vegetables, meats and snacks and start comparing prices. Do the math and see if you can start substituting some organic items for non-organic items. For example, if you were buying 5 apples, 1 pound of chicken, 2 pounds of steak, and some starches (like potatoes or rice) for around $30 per week, see how much you can get at the organic market for the same total cost, and make some adjustments. Perhaps you

could purchase more chicken and less steak, since poultry is generally cheaper than beef. Don't hesitate to make these changes as the health of your body depends on it.

3. Commit to making a complete shift in shopping habits and routine after the first week. As you rid your kitchen of all the foods with chemicals and start adding healthier options to your diet, you'll find there's no turning back! You'll be enjoying tastier food and feeling more energetic than ever before.

Let's move on to learn the next step in empowering your body.

<u>Chapter 3</u>:

Fueling the Body

Outdated Eating Machine

Your body is an incredible sacred machine and should be treated with the utmost respect. Most of us eat too much or eat too late at night, and quite frankly, this becomes strenuous on our internal organs.

No matter who you are, it's likely that you or someone you know has a weight problem. This is mostly attributed to the increased consumption of energy dense foods, such as soda, candy, and prepackaged foods.

The combination of dangerous processed-foods and an overall lack of self-control over how much food our body ingest are the main causes of the obesity epidemic.

Our bodies were not designed to handle food the way we do today—from eating solely for survival to eating simply whenever we feel like it.

So, what can you do to make sure you don't follow this gluttonous path?

You must learn to control how much you eat and change up what you eat for every meal, such as eating the right amounts of fruits and vegetables every day which will not only save you from chronic diseases but will keep your body happy.

The One-Third Meal Plan

Let's go through a plan to add more vegetables and fruits to your meal and exercise portion control. It is based on establishing the following:

- **Base**: The recommended amount of food type per meal. For example, in one meal you may have a fruit, a vegetable, a meat, some dairy, and whatever condiments that may go with it. For beverages, focus on including water and natural fruit juices. If you use sweeteners, stick with the unrefined sweeteners, like molasses, honey, or maple syrup.

- **Routine**: A fixed schedule in which we do things, such as eating dinner at the same time every day, waking up at the same time, etc. Come up with a schedule of when meals should begin and end each day.

- **Portioning**: How you will organize the ingredients you've chosen as your base at meal time. For example, since we want to maximize consumption of fruits and vegetables, then that portion should cover half of your plate.

When putting this into practice, remember that this is not a diet, but rather a way to eat better so that you can empower your body, have more energy, and feel better about yourself.

Now here's how you will combine the three:

1. Set up your base by choosing different kinds of vegetables, fruits, meats (white and red), etc., and your beverages. Be sure to include lots of water and 100% natural juices.

2. Your meals should be well-spaced, so that you don't put too much stress on your digestive system. These organs normally process food and distribute nutrients throughout your body quite efficiently, but when bombarded with too much sugar or fat they are forced to work overtime. Eventually, they will be so worn out

that they will allow toxins into your bloodstream, leading to fatigue, body odor, and an increased susceptibility to health issues. By spacing out meals further apart, for instance, three or four hours apart, it allows our digestive system to more easily break down our food. It's also important to stop eating after a specific time at night, usually eight or nine. This gives our bodies sufficient time to process the last meal before bed.

3. "Make it right" by using the portion method. The portion method consists of dividing your plate in three, where you will organize the food that makes up your base.

- For breakfast: Fill half of your plate with various fruits. The remaining half is divided in two. Choose a starch for one of the sections, such as toast, or a pancake. The remaining quarter can be filled with another healthy choice such as eggs. When having cereal, fill your bowl only a third full, add milk to fill another third, and then top with a generous portion of fruit, such as strawberries or blueberries.

- For lunch or dinner: Make sure that half of your plate is made up of vegetables, a quarter is made up of starches and the remaining quarter for meat.

- For snacks: Try using your hands to measure portions. For example, if you like snacking on nuts, measure out a serving in the palm of your hands. The same can be done with vegetables or fruits. Your goal should be to have at least 5 palm-sized servings of fruits and vegetables a day. So eating these as snacks is an excellent way to meet your daily goal.

- For beverages: Water should be your primary drink of choice as it is recommended that you drink 8 glasses of water per day, which is a lot! However, when you do choose to drink other beverages, only fill your glass two-third's full. This will ensure you do not bombard your body with too much sugar. When adding sugar to beverages like coffee, try substituting brown for white. White sugar is highly-processed, so brown sugar is a better alternative or try natural sweeteners.

Portion Eating

Now, to really see how it works, let's illustrate this method with an example of how this could work in your own life.

Early in the morning you start your day with breakfast. Let's say that you decide you want to eat cereal today topped with berries. So, you fill a third of your bowl with cereal and another third with milk. Use your hand to measure a serving (or two) of berries to top your cereal. If you would like a glass of juice or coffee, fill two-third's of your glass and, if necessary, sweeten your coffee with brown or agave sugar.

Around noon, you move on to lunch, where you'd like to eat a balanced meal of chicken, peas and rice. Using the portioning method, you would select foods from your base items list and then organize them the following way; 50% of your plate is filled with peas, 25% chicken, and 25% rice. This way you eat more vegetables, less meat, and less starch. Portioning your lunch this way will allow your digestive system to process food efficiently.

Now on to in-between meal time, your afternoon snack. Why include a snack? Eating a healthy snack will ensure your body is adequately fueled to make it to dinner time. Skipping this important light meal will likely lead to over-indulgence at dinner. So take the time to eat a snack, making sure that the amount you take fits in the palm of your hand.

Finally there is dinner. This final meal of the day is eaten in the evening, making sure it is finished no later than 9 pm. Fill your plate half full with steamed broccoli and carrots, 25% with fish and 25% with mashed potatoes. You've successfully put together a nutritious dinner without much thought. Choose water as your beverage or fill a glass two-third's full of juice or soda, whichever you prefer.

Note that instead of counting calories—which can easily become exhausting and confusing—you are simply making more space on your plate for fruits and vegetables, while at the same time placing limitations on the amount of meat and starches you eat throughout the day.

Exercise: Update Eating Machine

Now, it's your turn. Follow the guidelines to establish your base, set your routine and start portioning.

1. Set up your base by following the healthy eating rule—include a variety of vegetables, fruits, meats and fish, starches and beverages.

2. Set a schedule for eating meals. Your meals should be every 3-4 hours and choose a stop time. Create your timeline however you wish to meet your own personal schedule.

3. Practice portioning your meals and beverages by organizing your plate. Half of your plate should be for fruits and vegetables while the rest is divided between meats and starches. Don't forget to drink 8 glasses of water per day.

<u>Chapter 4:</u>

Exercising the Body

Workout Simplified

Almost every day we are bombarded with messages from different sources, like magazines that make claims like, "Lose ten pounds in ten days!" or "Six-pack abs in six moves!" It seems that people's exercise routines change constantly—it's no wonder most of us get confused and want to throw our hands up in defeat.

To simplify it all for you, keep this in mind, as long as the physical activity you make makes you sweat, you are burning calories and stimulating vital hormones like adrenaline.

Professionals like Dr. Esther M. Steinberg point out that adrenaline improves your memory and stimulates your metabolism throughout the day. According to Dr. Steinberg, a single adrenaline burst—which lasts for only a moment—can heighten your senses and spur you into action immediately.

The best way to stimulate secretion of this hormone is through regular exercise.

Types of Exercises

There are so many types of exercise, all of which are beneficial. Here are some options to consider adding to your daily routine:

- **Aerobics**: This type of workout works all the parts of your body and is a great method to burn fat fast. You'll follow a specific routine while engaging your muscles and practicing rhythmic breathing. Examples include swimming, biking, and running.

- **Cardio**: Exercises, like running or even walking, to make you sweat and stay in shape. You might be wondering—what's the difference between aerobic and cardio? They're practically the same, but aerobic is meant for increasing oxygen-intake for stronger lungs while cardio targets in strengthening the heart, hence, cardiovascular exercise.

- **Pilates**: A group of exercises where you adopt certain poses for a brief period of time that stretch your muscles and strengthen your body. It is excellent for improving posture and muscle tone.

- **Yoga**: Yoga is an ancient Hindu practice, but today it is widely popular for general health and relaxation that uses simple meditation and breathing control while stretching to increase blood flow and improve flexibility.

- **Weightlifting**: The sport or exercise of lifting barbells or other weights. It's good for strengthening muscles and toning the body.

- **Other alternatives**: There are a lot of other ways to get exercise, including dancing, playing a sport like basketball or football, cleaning the house or just horsing around with your kids.

Any amount of exercise is better than no exercise, so don't let time constraints keep you from exercising. You can work out for as long as you wish. However, be aware that the timing of exercise can make a big difference in terms of burning calories. Your goal should be 20 minutes at a minimum and an hour maximum.

You'll need to establish a reasonable frequency for your workouts, depending on your schedule. Working out a few times per week is good, but to maximize the benefits of exercise your goal should be 3 times a week at a minimum.

When developing your exercise plan, keep in mind is that you can work out whatever time of day you choose. For most of us, that means working out either first thing in the morning or at night to accommodate work or school schedules.

The absolute best time to exercise is in the morning, as you'll reap the benefits throughout the day. Thanks to a post-workout adrenaline rush, your body will be enhanced, your overall mood with be elevated and you will feel empowered to make the most of your day.

However, morning exercise is not for everyone. Remember that any amount of exercise, at any time of day, is better than no exercise. If you choose to work out in the evening, try to do it early enough that the adrenaline rush will wear off a bit before you go to bed.

Physical Activities Schedule

Now the most important question is; what type of exercise should you go for?

Quite simply, pick whatever works for you. What activities do you enjoy doing? The more enjoyable the exercise, the more likely you are to stick with it. To keep it interesting, combine 3 to 4 disciplines per week that will make up a diverse "workout package."

Now let's put these suggestions to work:

1. Pick a minimum of 3 disciplines; for example, cardio, yoga and aerobics.

2. Decide on timing, duration and frequency. For instance, you choose to work out in the morning (to take advantage of the benefits of adrenaline), for 30 minutes 4 times a week, because you want to lose weight and feel good about yourself.

3. The last step is to create and implement your plan, which in this example could look like this:

i. Cardio every Monday for 30 minutes
ii. Yoga for 30 minutes every Tuesday morning
iii. Aerobics every Wednesday morning for 30 minutes
iv. Cardio every Thursday morning for 30 minutes

So with this example, you've met all your goals; the frequency is 4 times a week, duration is 30 minutes per day and the timing is every morning.

Note that the location of your workouts is wherever you are most comfortable. You can workout at home, at the gym, at a park or swimming pool. To add variety, you can workout at different locations throughout the week. It doesn't matter because it's about doing what works best for you.

Exercise: Choose Workouts

Now it's your turn!

Using these guidelines, set up a plan that works for you to start empowering your body. Follow step one by choosing a minimum of 3 disciplines, then move onto step two by choosing timing (morning or night), duration (from 20 minutes up to an hour), and frequency (minimum 3 times a week). Then it's time to implement your plan.

After the first week, complete the following evaluation:

- How do you feel, a week after you've started your new exercise schedule?

- Describe how you feel your body is being empowered? (Do you still feel tired or do you feel more motivated?)

Chapter 5:

Rejuvenating the Body

Recharge Session

Now that you've learned how you should eat and how you should exercise to greater empower your body, it's time to learn how to best rest the right way. A good night's sleep is associated with a host of health benefits, such as immune system strengthening and better pain recovery, so it is imperative we make it a priority.

Though we often fall short, the recommended amount of sleep for an adult is between 7 and 8 hours of sleep every day. This amount of sleep allows you to rest enough so that your body can regenerate itself and allow you to be more focused and more energized the next day.

You should go to bed every night at the same time. The ideal bedtime is different for everyone, but it's usually around 9:00 or 10:00 pm. Depending on when you naturally (or have to) get up, this may change. The earlier you have to get up, the earlier you should go to bed.

If you don't get enough sleep, you can try to catch up on sleep during the day by taking naps. Short naps have been found to rejuvenate the mind and body. Oftentimes though we feel really tired, we only need a short rest.

Pre-SLEEP-Quisites

To get that great night's sleep you've been yearning for, you need set the stage for sleep.

How should we get ready for bed? As in, how do we prepare for a good night sleep? According to experts like

Charles Linden, there are things that can be done throughout the day or before bed to prepare our body for a good night sleep.

Let's go through a list of four simple rules that are sure to have you sleeping better in no time:

RULE 1: **Be more active during the day.** Move around! If you have a job in which you sit a lot, periodically get up and walk around. Take the stairs. Park far away from the office. Take a walk on your lunch break. Exercise when you get home.

RULE 2: **Take a hot bath before bed.** The warm water will comfort you while your muscles relax. Warm water actually signals our body to start producing melatonin, the hormone that induces sleep. After you are done, you will feel more at ease and ready for deep, restorative sleep.

<u>RULE 3</u>: **Find simple ways to relax.** There are a variety of activities we can do to relax to prepare for bed. Aromatherapy, the use of aromatic plant extracts or essential oils in massage or baths in order to alter one's mood, is very popular. We use aromatherapy for the purpose of altering our cognitive, psychological or physical well-being.

<u>RULE 4</u>: **Stretch before bed.** Your body goes through a lot in the course of day. You use your legs and feet to walk and exercise, your fingers and hands to type, write and carry things, and your brain to think and solve problems. That is a lot of work! As you age, these activities become more difficult. Joint pain can prevent you from sleeping well. The best thing you can do to remedy this is to stretch your muscles before bed.

Just by following four simple rules, you will be amazed by how easily you can achieve total relaxation. Your body will be rejuvenated and you'll have forgotten all about that hard day at work. You will also find it easy to go to bed at 10 pm and fall asleep quickly.

Applying the Rules of Sleep

Let's go through an example to see how you can effectively manage these rules:

1. Find creative ways to stay active throughout your day. For example, instead of asking your coworker to bring you a file, get up and go get it. Or if you are teaching your son to read and you need to change the book you are reading, instead of asking him to go get it, do it yourself. Get moving like that during the day and your body will shut down (not in the real sense) by 10 pm.

2. Relax after work. If your schedule won't allow for a massage service, do it yourself with the following exercise:

Sitting on a chair, slowly rotate your elbows from front to back, 10 times. Then, do the same with your neck. Slowly rotate your neck left to right. Use your hands to gently squeeze the muscle between you neck and shoulder. Hold for a moment, then release. Use your fingers to apply pressure to any sore spots in your neck and shoulders.

3. Try a warm bath in the evening. Allow yourself to relax while you soak for at least 30 minutes. You can also incorporate aromatherapy and message therapy as mentioned previously. For example, you could take a bath with a few drops of lavender oil, or give yourself a massage with rose oil.

4. Stretch your upper body with the following exercise:

Raise both arms into the air and join your hands together. Extend your palms upward as if you were trying to touch the ceiling. Then, rotate your torso each way 5 times. Then form a C-shape with your upper body by flexing your spine backwards.

This example illustrates how to use each of the rules to promote better sleep and empower your body.

Now, it's your turn to experiment with these rules.

Just remember, get busy during the day and then find ways to relax and unwind before bed. It really is that simple!

After you've tried these suggestions, re-evaluate the quality of your sleep, your mood and your overall performance the following day. The difference will be remarkable!

Chapter 6:

Redesigning the Body

Now that we have gone over your trainings to total body empowerment, it's up to you to continue this path—but not before we give you your final exercises.

Exercise 1: Know Organic

Complete the following quiz to see how much you know about organic food.

1. What category of food is sold in large quantities?

a.) Cheap chemically-enhanced food.

b.) Fruits and veggies.

c.) Exotic fruits.

d.) Organic food.

2. What is the difference between organic and non-organic food?

a.) Organic food is grown under more controlled conditions.

b.) Organic food is also grown with pesticides and other harmful chemicals, but at a lesser amount.

c.) Organic food is brought from overseas while non-organic food is produced in America.

d.) Organic food is more bland in taste.

3. What types of problems might you get by eating GMO food?

a.) You are more sensitive to inflammations.

b.) You are more likely to develop cancer or suffer from hormonal imbalances.

c.) You are more prone to cavities.

d.) You are more at risk of obesity.

(Answers: 1 is a, 2 is a, and 3 is b)

Exercise 2: Upgrade Meals

Follow the guidelines on portion control to come up with your own personal plan for healthy eating for three days.

Create your base, by selecting the type of veggies, meats, fruits, cereals, starches, and beverages you will eat. Next, create your daily routine for how many meals you will eat and how often. And finally, organize your portions by making more space on your plate for fruits and vegetables while at the same time placing limitations on the amount of meat and starches you will eat.

After 3 days, evaluate how you feel. In what ways has this change in your diet empowered your body?

Exercise 3: Get Physical

Get physical by doing the following exercise:

1. Lie on your back and slowly start pedaling as if you were on a bicycle. Make sure your movements are slow and controlled. After 3 minutes you will start to feel as if your legs are becoming heavier. If you are able, try to go for another 2 minutes before resting. Repeat three more times.

2. Next, keeping your legs straight, lift your legs straight up in the air. Then slowly lower them down without touching the floor. Do this in 5 series of ten, resting in between. You will feel this exercise strengthening your abdominal muscles.

3. Lastly, run in place for 15 minutes. You will start sweating and feel a release of adrenaline.

Evaluate your state of mind after this exercise. Are you in a better mood? Explain.

How does your body feel? Do you feel lighter? Do you feel you could push yourself to do more the next day? Explain.

Exercise 4: Prepare Rest

Before bed, do the following stretching exercise:

1. Lie on your back, with both your arms stretched above your head. Breathe in and out, slowly 10 times.

2. Bring your left knee to your chest (holding it firmly) to your chest. Do the same thing with the other leg (5 times).

3. Bring both knees to your chest and count to 10.

4. Sit back up and try to touch your toes with your hands. Keep that position for 20 seconds. Then, release your toes.

5. Roll your shoulders backward 5 times and loosen your neck joints by circling your neck 3 times clockwise, then 3 times again the other way.

When done, head to bed.

The next day, evaluate your experience. Did stretching help you relax and fall asleep faster? Did you experience less joint pain?

Chapter 7:

Embracing the Powerful Body

Bodily Neglect

The many benefits of body empowerment are undeniable. A healthy body quite simply leads to a happier life. And who couldn't use a little more happiness?

Too often people believe money is the way to find happiness. Our work occupies our attention and we neglect to give thought to what we put on our plates and how we prioritize sleep and exercise. As a result, our body suffers.

Part of the weight problem in society today is that many people don't have as much time to work out and eat right as they have work, families, and other obligations that take up much of their time. People want something that's quick and easy. We live in comfy insulated boxes with a wide access to various foodstuffs that couldn't be unhealthier for us.

There's a lot working against us in the modern world, but we CAN fight back against it. We need to realize this and actively change, if we really want to live healthier.

Bodily Perfect

Body empowerment is about mutually respecting your body, feeding your body what it needs and paying close attention to your overall health. Take care of your body, and it will take care of you.

Incorporating organic food into your diet is one of the best ways to eat your way to a healthier body. With a little thoughtful consideration and budgeting, it is possible to make the switch to organic, at least in part. Reducing the consumption of processed foods is critical to promoting a healthier body.

Staying mindful of portion sizes and focusing on eating more vegetables and fruits is a simple and easy way to eat better without expending time and resources on confusing diet programs.

Exercise and rest are also essential, given our stressful—yet mostly sedentary—lifestyle. Our bodies were meant to move, so keep yours active! No amount of exercise is too little. Make time in the evenings for relaxation before bed, and prioritize sleep. Your body needs to recuperate after a stressful day.

If you want a stronger, healthier, more agile body tomorrow, start empowering your body TODAY!

Body Empowerment

Body Empowerment

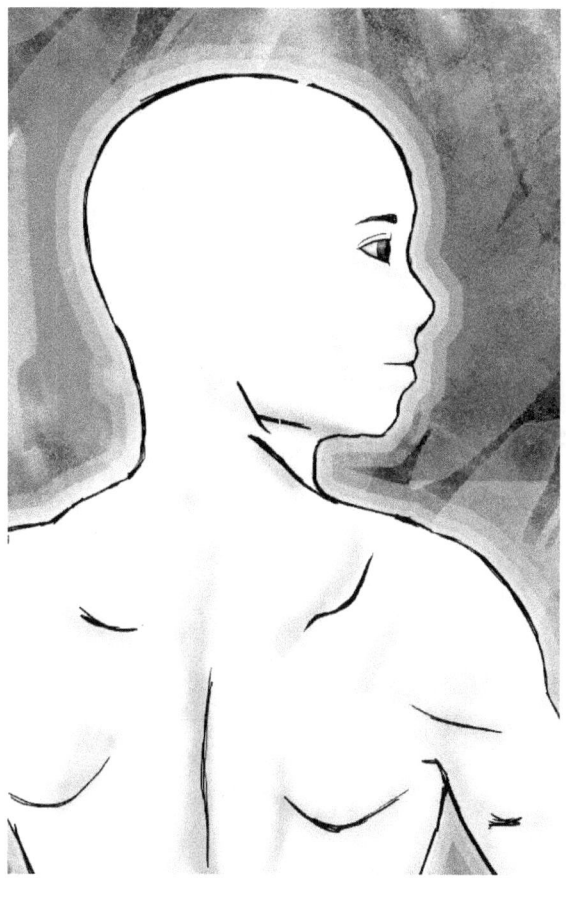

Body Empowerment